Eyegames

Easy and Fun Visual Exercises

An Occupational Therapist and Optometrist
Offer Activities to Improve Vision!

D1115815

Lois Hickman, MS, OTR, FAOTA
Rebecca E. Hutchins, OD, FCOVD

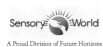

A Proud Division of Future Horizons

All marketing and publishing rights guaranteed to and reserved by
Sensory World, 1010 N. Davis Dr., Arlington, TX 76012.

Sensory World
info@sensoryworld.com
www.sensoryworld.com
(877) 775-8968
(682) 558-8941
(682) 558-8945 (fax)

1st edition ©2000 Belle Curve Records, Inc
2nd edition ©2002 Sensory Resources, LLC
3rd edition ©2010 Sensory World

Printed in the USA

It is the responsibility of the user of these materials to ensure that all
activities are conducted with appropriate supervision. Exercise due care
in selecting activities for a particular individual, especially with respect to
safety, developmental level, and age appropriateness. We recommend that
you consult with qualified health professionals regarding interventions.

Cover design: Composure Graphics
Illustrator: Lynda Farrington Wilson

ISBN-13: 978-1-935567-17-2

Table of Contents

Introduction

The development of healthy visual perception requires two basic elements:

The presence of light (with sunlight being the standard)

A strong integration of all of the body's sensory experiences

Sight, sound, touch, and smell, as well as balance and movement (vestibular sense) and muscle control (proprioceptive sense), all contribute to visual perception. All of these senses were developed on our planet, which is governed by gravity and is perpetually in the presence of sunlight. Experiencing life out-of-doors, in relationship to the natural world, is our heritage, whether we are a child or an adult, a therapist, or a client. Our health and the health of Earth depends upon our honoring and acting on this connection.

Vision therapists and occupational therapists recognize a common ground in their understanding of the visual aspects of sensory integration and sensory processing. These therapies can complement each other, yielding a more comprehensive approach to treatment and education.

Eyegames is the result of the work and collaboration of two renowned therapists—Lois Hickman, MS, OTR, FAOTA; and Rebecca Hutchins, OD, FCOVD. This book and the activities contained within are based in therapeutic theory and practice but are also designed to be fun and educational. Both Lois and Rebecca support the well-proven philosophy that learning is much easier when it's fun! They each live on small backyard farms with a variety of animals, yet both have worked in the inner city. They have collaborated on a summer camp for developmentally delayed children. They stress that any activity must be open to change in response to the need of the client or the moment. It's important to let go of preconceived ideas and allow your ideas to take flight to fully benefit from these activities. After all, therapy can be seen as a dance between therapist and client. Furthermore, activities done in the natural world, under the sun, may provide the most benefit.

Each of these fields—occupational therapy and behavioral optometry—contributes to the philosophies inherent in this book. A clear understanding of the differences between these fields will help you grasp the overlap and strengthen your comprehension of the activities and ideas presented in *Eyegames*.

Behavioral Optometrist's Viewpoint

The behavioral model of vision began with the work of Dr A. M. Skeffington in the 1920s. This quote from Dr Skeffington expresses the core philosophy of behavioral optometry:

> *Vision cannot be separated from the total individual or from any other sensory systems, as it is integrated in all of human performance. Vision is learned, and therefore, trainable. Many visual problems appear to be triggered by environmental factors. They may be developmental or stress induced. Behavioral optometrists put a major emphasis on the prevention of vision problems as well as enhancing visual related performance which is at a level less than the individual's potential.*

Occupational Therapist's Viewpoint

From its beginnings in the early 1900s, occupational therapy has exemplified the conviction that purposeful activity (occupation) is a pivotal element in human life. Quoting a 1979 statement from the American Occupational Therapy Association:

> *Man is an active being whose development is influenced by purposeful activity. Using their capacity for intrinsic motivation, human beings are able to influence their physical and mental health and their social and physical environment through purposeful activity. Human life includes a process of continuous adaptation. Adaptation is a change in function that promotes survival and self-actualization. The field of occupational therapy emphasizes three equally important elements in life: self-care, work, and play.*

The activities in *Eyegames* reflect these philosophies. They are purposeful, applicable to daily life, and playful. May you enjoy and benefit from the wealth of information gathered here!

The information contained in this book was created out of the imagination and creativity of therapists and clients. It is not meant to give every idea possible for exploration in any area—it is meant to stimulate creativity and collaboration. It is not meant to be used as a recipe book! It is not intended as medical advice, as a means of diagnosing visual problems, or as a substitute for optometric vision therapy or occupational therapy. Please see the definition of optometric vision therapy (page 21), which explains that it includes the use of lenses, prisms, filters, occlusion, and other equipment and is performed with the direct supervision of an optometrist. Even the home-based activities included here, which fall under the umbrella of occupational therapy, are best done after consulting with an occupational therapist.

The intent of this book is informational and educational. Always consult a healthcare professional should the need for one arise. We strongly recommend regular eye examinations from your eye doctor. We also recommend consultation with your behavioral optometrist or occupational therapist if there are difficulties with vision or with sensory integration.

The Development of Vision

Vision is founded on the basic senses, ontogenetically (the predictable way babies are expected to develop, based on centuries of observation) and phylogenetically (the way human beings have developed as a species over time). Vision began as a life-saving distance receptor for land animals, in the presence of light. It became increasingly complex as the brain became more complex, as it connected with all the various senses and with emotion and memory. It has become finely tuned, evolving into a sophisticated form of perception. The visual areas of the brain are strongly dependent on touch for proper development. When a person encounters stress or trauma, vision can revert to its primitive alerting, life-saving function.

To feel the interconnectedness of vision with the bodily experiences of vibration, movement, pressure, smell, and touch, take the time to slowly imagine the sense of touching:

- Velvet
- Rabbit fur
- A rose petal
- Snow
- A kitten
- Sticky syrup
- A pretzel
- A razor blade

Did you reach for or recoil from touching each one? Were there emotions or memories associated with your reactions?

Now imagine:

- Walking through mud
- Skiing
- Rolling in leaves

- Sky-diving
- An icy-cold shower
- Walking on the moon
- Jumping off a roof
- Rowing a boat
- Sliding on grease
- A bear hug
- A boa constrictor
- Braiding a horse's mane

Where in your body did you feel sensations as you visualized them?

Now, close your eyes and imagine spelling the name of:

- Your favorite dessert
- Your favorite flower
- A jungle animal
- A friend's name
- A foreign country
- Your childhood address

If you were unable to visualize some things on the list, was it because you had never experienced them? It is far easier to visualize what we have already experienced.

Visual learning starts very early in life. From birth, a baby lays the foundation for understanding the many aspects of vision: What is up and down, and what is diagonal, horizontal, or vertical? What is close, and what is far away? Is something soft or hard, rough or smooth, hot or cold? All of this must first be experienced through touch and then associated with visual interpretation. Additionally, how the primary caregivers choose to move a child about (slings, infant carriers, or backpacks) has a huge impact on the child's understanding of directionality and gravity, which also plays a part in vision development.

As a baby develops more and more independence in balance and movement, he is freer to explore the environment and refine the relationships between spatial and tactile experiences. Most children develop vision in well-documented stages.

In utero, even before birth, there are strong pulsing sounds and vibrations. There is little light, if any, and the senses of hearing and touch are better developed than sight at birth. For 9 months, the baby lives in a water world—warm, embracing, and comforting.

Birth to 7 Weeks

Newborns are fascinated with light and patterns. Their sight is nurtured by light. Recognition of the pattern of the caregiver's face is clearest within a narrow range: an 8-inch distance from the baby's face. Objects beyond that distance are a blur, and the newborn has much more awareness of movement than of form. The baby desires and needs touch, cuddling, movement, and the soothing voice of the caregiver. The security of being cared for is critical.

2 to 4 Months

The baby begins developing basic eye-hand coordination and depth perception. Babies enjoy shaking rattles, grabbing and exploring objects, and holding and mouthing soft toys. They also find joy in the baby jokes of peek-a-boo, pat-a-cake, and other early games they play with the people who love them.

5 to 8 Months

The baby begins establishing general muscle control, and sometime around 8 months, will start creeping and exploring on his own. His visual field extends out farther, from 10 to 24 inches. Fine-motor movements are more refined and purposeful, enabling the exploration of small objects. Control of ocular muscles is part of this general muscular development, and this control should stop any early crossing or drifting of his eyes.

9 to 18 Months

The baby can see up to 4 feet away. Many infants test their walking skills, using a wide base of support, with arms up in "high-guard" position. They gradually walk more freely, with arms down and hands free. By 18 months, babies develop the skill to walk sideways and backwards and to stand on one foot. The baby explores a variety of shapes and textures, combines objects into towers, and puts objects in containers. He may even try to imitate a scribble.

19 to 36 Months

The visual field extends out from 4 to 10 feet, and peripheral awareness gradually extends farther, as well. Development progressively leads toward being able to run, jump, kick, and catch. Fine-motor control also expands, and with it the ability to place simple puzzle pieces, take the caps off bottles, imitate pencil strokes, and dress more independently.

3 Years and Older

A 3-year-old child can see up to 10 to 16 feet away, and a 4-year-old can see a distance of 16 to 20 feet. By the time a child is 5 years old, he or she has wide peripheral vision, in addition to 20-foot depth perception. The typical 5-year-old child can use scissors and paper clips, fold paper, tie an overhand knot, button small buttons, and color within lines much of the time. The preceding timetables and the following passage were taken from Kavner's *Your Child's Vision: A Parent's Guide to Seeing, Growing, and Developing:*

> *Visual exploration is vital as the child matures and becomes ready for the classroom experience. This visual exploration has encompassed motor development, visual motor development, expansion of personal and social space to include others, three-dimensional space, going from nurturing to independent space, and the development of increased peripheral awareness.*

In about 5 years, a child's development progresses from use of vision at near distances and with basic body movements to use of vision at both near and far distances and with more refined, controlled body

Once a child begins school, an estimated 80% of all classroom learning takes place through the visual pathways.

movement skills. The child becomes increasingly able to embrace the world visually and socially. This early development provides the foundation for learning and developing other life skills.

By the time a child is ready to attend school, the basic senses of movement and touch have blended with vision. Integrating the senses of movement, touch, and vision allows us to visualize experiences. Imagine the sensation of using your hands to scrape the seeds from a pumpkin, looking down from the top of a tall building or mountain, watching a speeding train, or racing up a flight of stairs. Imagine the sensation of writing your name with chalk on a sidewalk. Imagine how to spell the name of your favorite flower or animal or dessert. Most of these images integrate vision with other sensory experiences.

Problems with Visual Perception

Any interference with basic sensory pathways, or inefficient integration of these senses with vision, can cause difficulty with learning any task. Even a child with perfect eyesight may suffer from severe visual difficulties that can affect academic, athletic, or daily life performance.

Even mild difficulties can cause problems. Most children are born with healthy eyes and neurological structures. They are able to integrate all the basic senses—touch, movement, hearing, and balance—with their visual experiences. They learn to judge distance, the movement of objects in relation to their bodies, and even the texture, size, and weight of objects "just by looking." Visual performance is dependent on the relationship between visual movement skill, body movement skill, and tactile perception.

Children with visual problems may not have had the touch, movement, and motor experiences that form the foundation for normal visual performance, or they may not have been able to integrate these experiences because of an underlying sensory processing issue. Problems with visual perception may result from complex issues of sensory processing or may primarily result from visual interpretation issues. Whatever the reason, children with visual difficulties are frequently mislabeled as having behavior or attention problems or being underachievers or slow learners.

According to the Web site of the College of Optometrists in Vision Development, the certifying body for behavioral optometrists, typical symptoms of visual difficulties include:

Physical signs or symptoms

- Frequent headaches or eye strain
- Blurring of distance or near vision, particularly after reading or other close work
- Avoidance of close work or other visually demanding tasks
- Poor judgment of depth

- Turning of an eye in or out, up or down
- Tendency to cover or close one eye, or favor the vision in one eye
- Double vision
- Poor hand-eye coordination
- Difficulty following a moving target
- Dizziness or motion sickness

Performance problems

- Poor reading comprehension
- Difficulty copying information from one place to another (as in hand-copying or typing)
- Loss of place, repetition, and/or omission of words while reading
- Difficulty changing focus from distance vision to near vision and back
- Poor posture when reading or writing
- Poor handwriting
- Can respond orally but can't get the same information down on paper
- Letter and word reversals
- Difficulty judging sizes and shapes

When one or more of these symptoms is present, consult a behavioral optometrist to determine whether glasses, contact lenses, or vision therapy might be necessary. In the presence of motor-based performance problems or difficulty in posture, however, poor handwriting, fear of movement, or spatial disorientation indicate the need for an evaluation by an occupational therapist who has been specially trained in evaluating and treating sensory processing disorders, or SPDs— see *www.spdfoundation.net* for further information. On the other hand, a child who is initially seen by an occupational therapist may not exhibit difficulty in sensory integration, and the therapist may then refer the child to a behavioral optometrist; of course, many times, children benefit best from participating in both types of therapy.

When a child receives the appropriate intervention, at the right time, significant progress will be seen.

When making an appointment with an eye doctor, the Optometric Extension Program Foundation (a nonprofit organization dedicated to vision education) recommends that you ask the following questions:

- Do you offer a full series of near-point visual tests?
- Do you provide vision care and vision therapy in your office? If not, do you refer to a doctor who does?
- Do you administer academically related visual perception tests?
- Will you schedule another appointment during the year to check on progress?

When treating people with vision problems, behavioral optometrists use a complex program of activities that is tailored specifically for each person. Specific treatment can help with a wide range of problems, including:

- Traumatic brain injury
- Visual problems related to autism
- Visual problems resulting from cerebral palsy
- Stroke and other neuromuscular disorders
- Learning disabilities
- Strabismus (crossed or wandering eye)
- Amblyopia (lazy eye)

Treatment may eliminate the need for surgery or may enhance its effectiveness if surgery is necessary.

"A recent American Optometric Association survey of 1,001 respondents found that adults far underestimate how frequently children have vision problems, with nearly 90 percent unaware that 25% of children have some sight issues. According to the association, studies indicate that as many as 60% of children identified as "problem learners" actually have undetected vision problems that may be stunting their academic development."

— Rhonda Bodfield, "Vision Problems Can Be a Source of Kids' Bad Grades," *Arizona Daily Start,* September 2, 2009.

" Good vision does much more than simply enable a person to see the traffic lights when crossing the street or what a teacher is writing on the board. It helps him to lead a fully dimensional life with all the depth of understanding, breadth of feeling, and height of experience that this implies. Seeing, more than any other sense, guides and shapes a person's behavior and experience of life. You can understand then why I emphasize the importance of good vision, as it is one gift all people deserve.

Beyond the realm of medical or learning problems, behavioral optometry can help improve academic and athletic performance. A behavioral optometrist may prescribe lenses to help general visual functioning beyond improving visual acuity. Every 8 inches is a new visual field. Lenses that are needed to see a chalkboard across the room may not be the right lenses for working on the computer or for reading. "

— Richard Kavner, OD, FAAO

Vision and Autism

Rebecca E. Hutchins, OD, FCOVD

Look Me in the Eye is the title of a recent best-selling memoir of John Robison; the subtitle is, *My Life with Asperger's.* The book cover depicts a small boy with his eyes squeezed tightly shut. The prologue begins, "Look me in the eye, young man," and the author proceeds to explain how his inability to do so was consistently interpreted to mean that he "was just no good." He then admits that to this day he "finds visual input to be distracting."

In this section, I will provide a description of this and other visual characteristics common in individuals on the autism spectrum and present methods of evaluation and treatment for these visual differences. In addition, I've included a list of professional, layperson, and fiction books for further reading.

What visual behaviors are seen in people within the autism spectrum? Avoidance of eye contact isn't the only common visual behavior among those in this population. So are:

- Seeking out visual input, like flashing or rotating lights
- Flicking hands and watching them
- Looking at something, then looking away before picking it up
- Peering out of the sides of the eyes
- Using peripheral rather than central vision for many activities

A paper on vision and autism published in October of 1997 by the College of Optometrists in Vision Development (the organization that certifies optometrists who provide vision therapy) states it succinctly: "Vision problems are very common in individuals with autism."

What is meant by the term *vision?* My favorite working definition is, "the deriving of meaning and the directing of action stimulated by light." Mull over this definition, and you'll see that determining whether or not a child can see 20/20 barely scratches the surface of exploring a child's experience of "vision." For this reason, although standard eye testing is important to treat or rule out diseases of the eye and assess the need for glasses to see clearly, it is not used to evaluate the ability of the child to use vision in learning and movement.

Who evaluates the derivation of meaning and directing of action, and what are the factors that are examined?

The field known as behavioral or developmental optometry is designed to evaluate the breadth of this visual spectrum. One way to explain some of the factors that are examined over and above the 20/20 criterion is use of the mnemonic device of the "Seven F's:"

- Following
- Fixation
- Focus
- Fusion
- Flexibility
- Field
- Fatigue

Let's go through the definitions of each of these important visual skills:

Following refers to actively moving both eyes in a smooth and coordinated movement to follow a moving object. When following is tested in the examination room, it is called *tracking* or *pursuits*. There is another type of self-directed, point-to-point eye movement—a saccade—that occurs when a child tries to navigate a maze or connect the dots. This, too, requires consistent, bilateral control of the eyes.

Fixation refers to the ability to hold both eyes centrally on an object. When reading, an individual must be able to fixate the word long enough to derive meaning.

Focus is necessary to see something clearly. When it is blurry, we say it is out of focus. The brain doesn't like blurring—it limits our abilities to derive meaning and take direct action.

Fusion is a technical term and means that (a) both eyes are aimed at the same place in space and (b) that the two images are melded into one (hopefully) three-dimensional object in the brain. If an individual has poor or no fusion, she may see two objects, or the world may appear flat and have no contour.

Flexibility of the visual system allows one to quickly and easily look back and forth in space and see clearly and singly.

Field refers to the full breadth of the limits of both eyes—up, down, right, and left. There can be organic, usually permanent field losses, but there can also be attentional, variable losses of visual field. For instance, when we are frightened, we have a tendency to attend only to what is right in front of us, limiting our field to a "tunnel" area. Using all of our visual field helps us to know where we are in space and where other people and objects are. It helps us to direct our actions.

Fatigue is a factor that can limit visual performance in many areas. If an individual with autism is very concentrated in using peripheral vision and ignores the central visual area (which is the opposite of how most people use their visual system), he may tire very quickly and not want to do tasks involving central vision.

Now that we've defined *vision* and how to evaluate it, what about autism? The visual system is usually the dominant form of learning and experience in the world. John Streff, an articulate behavioral optometrist, once said, "When vision is working well, it guides and leads; when it is not, it interferes."

Let's go back to the statement made by the College of Optometrists and Vision Development, "Vision problems are very common in individuals with autism." If this is the case, visual problems will interfere with a child's learning, ability to play sports, and daily life activities.

In individuals with autism, many of the distinct visual symptoms referred to previously occur for one of two reasons: either because "people with autism use visual information inefficiently" or because they "have hypersensitive vision and react by being visually defensive" (akin to tactile defensiveness). When a child is defensive to touch, she perceives it as dangerous and avoids it; likewise, to protect oneself from visual overwhelm and perceived danger, a child may look out of the sides of his eyes, and avoid direct visual confrontation. This occurs on a continuum, and a child with autism may show severe sensitivity and avoid experiences that other children may find interesting and nonthreatening.

What causes the visual problems related to autism, such as those cited previously in the bulleted list? The visual symptoms of autism can be explained by poor integration between the separate but equally necessary visual processing pathways: focal and ambient. The focal visual pathway gives information on what is being observed; the ambient one lets us know where we are and where an object is in space. Although it's an oversimplification, you could say that the focal system is the lead player in the derivation of meaning, while the ambient system takes the lead in directing action.

Those who work with individuals with autism, like Dr Melvin Kaplan, who wrote the book *Seeing through New Eyes: Changing the Lives of Children with Autism, Asperger Syndrome and other Developmental Disabilities through Vision Therapy,* explain that the vision problems "stem from deficits in the ambient vision processes involved in peripheral vision." As Dr Kaplan explains in his book,

"Autistic and other disabled children often have perfectly normal focal vision—the central vision that allows us to identify objects when we look straight at them—the problem lies instead with ambient vision, which involves the entire field of vision and tells us about the location of objects in space."

He goes on to explain, "Children with autism tend to look at other people from the corners of their eyes, not because they are aloof, but because monocular vision makes more sense than trying to interpret data from the two eyes that aren't working together. In addition, they may find it impossible to look at other people while conversing, because they can't process visual and auditory information at the same time." John Robison, author of *Look Me in the Eye,* and Temple Grandin, a well-known author and designer of animal research facilities, have both mentioned this in their books.

Dr Kaplan relates balance problems, walking on the toes, and difficulty interpreting space and time to a disordered ambient visual system. He and Drs Rose and Torgerson, who wrote an excellent comprehensive article entitled, "A Behavioral Approach to Vision and Autism," concur on the following two tools to be used to reeducate an individual to "organize space" and gain a stable periphery. (Behavioral optometrists explain that each individual creates his own visual world through coordination between the eyes and brain to interpret the environment through which the child moves. Recall that an autistic child has a disordered ambient system, which is what tells him where he is in space. Using the following activities gives the child different visual experiences and allows him to reexperience and thus redefine his relationship to the environment.)

The two tools used to reeducate an individual to "organize space" and gain a stable periphery are:

1. The introduction of yoked prism glasses
2. Participation in optometric vision therapy

To further elucidate these possibilities, descriptions of each follow.

Yoked prisms are lenses that are used to move the world in one direction— up, down, right, or left. The use of these lenses disrupts the ambient system and encourages reorganization and integration of ambient and focal vision. At times, the lenses are prescribed for full- or part-time wear outside of the office. Sometimes they are used as part of in-office vision therapy.

As I have worked with adults and children with many types of challenges, I have found that some activities are not as well suited to the autistic population. These individuals are frequently uncomfortable with relating in face-to-face interactions.

In working with children on the autism spectrum, I endeavor to make the activities fun, interesting, and noninvasive. As stated previously, lights and motion can be good attention-getters and can be used to direct focal involvement. One theory associated with social deficits in autism, the "mirror neuron theory," postulates that children with autism, unlike other children who possess mirror neurons, do not experience an activity themselves when they watch someone else perform it. I don't really know whether these children lack mirror neurons on not, but perhaps ironically, one tool I've found to be fascinating and fun in the vision therapy room is the use of a full-length mirror mounted on the wall or the back of a door. It seems that looking into a mirror is sometimes more acceptable for an autistic child than looking directly at an activity. The mirror allows one to see things at twice the distance and puts the individual and the room into context. Activities can be done while watching oneself perform in the mirror, or the mirror can be used as part of the activity—such as drawing glasses around your eyes and a mustache under your nose by using water-based markers right on the mirror surface. Looking at the surface of the mirror and then into the mirror

The official description of optometric vision therapy, as approved by the American Optometric Association, is:

An individualized treatment regimen prescribed for a patient in order to:
- Provide medically necessary treatment for diagnosed visual dysfunctions
- Prevent the development of visual problems
- Enhance visual performance to meet defined needs of the patient

Optometric vision therapy is appropriate treatment for visual conditions that include, but are not limited to:
- Strabismic and nonstrabismic binocular dysfunctions
- Amblyopia
- Accommodative dysfunctions
- Ocular motor dysfunctions
- Visual motor disorders
- Visual perceptual (visual information processing) disorders

The systematic use of lenses, prisms, filters, occlusion, and other appropriate materials, modalities, equipment, and procedures is integral to optometric vision therapy. The goals of the prescribed treatment regimen are to alleviate the signs and symptoms, achieve desired visual outcomes, meet the patient's needs and improve the patient's quality of life.

can also allow one to experience physiological diplopia, binocularity, and fusion. This description can hardly begin to describe the possibilities of using a mirror for enhancing, stabilizing, and expanding one's visual world.

This section is but a brief introduction to the ways in which a behavioral optometric evaluation can aid in the identification and treatment of some of the visual symptoms of autism. Eliminating or ameliorating some of the visual symptoms associated with autism can be a definitive step toward the stated vision therapy goal of "improving the patient's quality of life."

References

Rose M, Torgerson NG. A behavioral approach to vision and autism. *J Optom Vis Devel.* 1994;24:270.

Kaplan M. *Seeing through New Eyes: Changing the Lives of Children with Autism, Asperger Syndrome and Other Developmental Disabilities through Vision Therapy.* Philadelphia, PA: Jessica Kingsley Publishers; 2006:17.

Grandin T, Barron S. *Unwritten Rules of Social Relationships: Decoding Social Mysteries through the Unique Perspectives of Autism.* Arlington, TX: Future Horizons; 2005.

Additional Resources

Taub M, Russell R. Autism spectrum disorders: a primer for the optometrist. *Rev Optom.* 2007; 82-91.

Autism Spectrum Disorders and Cortical Visual Impairment: Two Worlds on Parallel Courses, Parts I and II. Presented at: Conference of the Association for Education and Rehabilitation of the Blind and Visually Impaired; July 2000; Denver, CO.

Look Me in the Eye: My Life with Asperger's, by John Robison

The Curious Incident of the Dog in the Night-time, by Mark Haddon

Speed of Dark, by Elizabeth Moon

Kantrowitz B, Scelfo B. Growing up with autism. *Newsweek.* November 27, 2006.

Biello D. Lack of Mirror neurons may help explain autism. *Sci Am.* December 5, 2005.

Guide to EyeGame Activities

Each of the following sections addresses a different vision therapy issue. We've created a series of treatment "games"—or "EyeGames"—to address these issues. Each EyeGame is explained and includes suggestions for variations.

All the EyeGames are coded in two ways: first, by an icon to indicate for which environmental settings they are most appropriate (ie, home, occupational therapy clinic, behavioral optometry clinic, school, or outdoors); and second, by the letter 'C" or "A" to indicate whether they are more appropriate for children or adults. However, all the children's activities could also be applicable for adults. It just depends on how game you are!

The following symbols and letters are used for quick reference:

Setting

 Home

 Occupational therapy or behavioral optometry clinic

 School

 Outdoors

Developmental Level

A Adult

C Child

EyeGame Activities

EyeGames should be performed *after* consultation with an optometrist or other appropriate eye care professional and an occupational therapist with training and experience in addressing sensory processing issues. Responsible adult supervision is essential to ensure the safety and effectiveness of these exercises.

Foundation Activities

Orienting to Light

Vision is not possible without light. We rarely acknowledge the importance of having the right quality of light and an adequate quantity of it. Sunlight is the light of our heritage, and it is the standard we judge all light by.

Children who seem unresponsive to their environment, who seldom reach for toys, can find reaching for light irresistible. Here are some suggestions for introducing light play with children with significant neurological or attentional issues. The following activities should be done in a dark or dimly lit area to ensure that focus is on the bowl of light, the light through the tunnel, the Lite Brite game, or the activities being done on the light table.

Nested Light

Use two large bowls, one nested inside the other. The inside bowl should be transparent. Place clear or colored nonblinking holiday lights between the two bowls, with textures or toys in the top bowl that you wish the child to reach for. Light invites the attention of sight, and the toys and textures invite the development of exploration in visual perception and eye-hand coordination.

Light through the Tunnel

Use nonblinking holiday lights that are enclosed in a plastic tube (you can buy them this way, already encased in tubing). These lights can be strung through play tunnels or large barrels to invite quadruped play activities, and toys can be scattered through the tunnel or hidden in pockets along the inside of the tunnels by using different kinds of closures, such as buttons, zippers, snaps, and Velcro.

Lite Brite ⌂ Ⓔ 🍎 **C**

This game, available at some toy stores (and sometimes at garage sales), contains a perforated panel with a light behind it and black paper in front. As a child places colored plastic pegs into the holes, a brightly colored picture or pattern emerges. It's really fun and beautiful in a darkened room. Follow specific patterns or create original ones. In the vision therapy clinic, red and green glasses are used to establish different input for each eye (one eye sees the lights as "red," the other as "green"— or sometimes described as "yellow-green").

For children who are attracted to light, introducing activities to them by using a light table (a glass-topped table lit from underneath) may be helpful before transitioning to activities that don't involve the use of light as an attraction. These are available commercially or can be made at home. Make sure that the table is safe and nonbreakable.

Orienting to Gravity

The vestibular and proprioceptive senses, which are linked to regulation of our movements and muscles, combine with vision to alert, stabilize, and focus our bodies. Movement and work by the large muscles prepare the body for skilled, fine-motor work. Eye muscles and big postural muscles should work together. As a child jumps, swings, and pushes, information from the vestibular and proprioceptive systems goes to all the muscles that have an effect on balance. These include the ocular—or eye— muscles. The child's body and eyes are alert and ready to work together.

With the strong foundation from the vestibular and proprioceptive senses, the tactile system combines with vision to enable discrimination and skill refinement. Accurate, discrete eye movements, combined with accurate, discrete tactile perception, make fine-motor control easier and more enjoyable.

Children and therapists cooperatively invented the following "foundation" activities. They provide a springboard for combining movement, muscles, touch, and vision within the realms of vision and occupational therapy. Many of these activities can be done outdoors, which gives our eyes the nourishment of light and the luxury of experiencing both near and far horizons—something that was once commonplace but is now all too rare! Whether children live in cities or suburbs, the amount of time spent in front of the TV or playing computer games, combined with the lack of outdoor space for freedom and creativity in play, all contribute to inadequate visual development. (For further information on this phenomenon, check out *The Last Child in the Woods,* by Richard Louv.)

Tic-Tac-Toe with Straws   C

Make a grid with tape on a carpet square, and use any shapes you like for the Xs and Os. The child could choose, draw, and cut out the lightweight paper shapes, which might be clouds and suns, stars and moons, or two different animals. Be sure the game surface is at least 8 inches off the floor, so that when the child kneels to play the game, posture and the visual distance to the game surface are optimized. The child will "pick up" the Xs and Os by sucking them up with the straw and placing them on the grid with a "puff." You can cut the straws to work efficiently and easily in the 8-inch distance.

Letter, Number, Word, and Shape Games with a Trampoline or Mat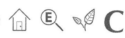

Draw letters and shapes on a trampoline with sidewalk chalk. The child can jump from one letter or shape to another. There are many variations you can create with this game:

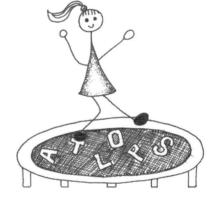

- Jump from one geometric shape to another in a preplanned order or as you or the child shouts it out.

- Jump from letter to letter to spell words. First, try to use the fewest number of jumps possible to spell each word. This takes big, bounding jumps! Then, to make the spelling more automatic, try to jump more quickly to spell words, requiring faster movement. You can even time this with a stopwatch, if the child thinks it would be fun to beat his own score.

- Have the child make up a phrase, then jump from letter to letter to spell all the words. For example, the child who helped create this game liked the phrase, "jumping fool."

- Print words around the trampoline. Jump from one word to another to create a sentence.

Downhill High-Speed Pick-up and Target Practice   C

This activity should be carefully graded and supervised to meet each child's individual needs. At first, you may need to help the child go down the ramp slowly, with the therapist controlling the speed.

Have the child lie on a scooter on his stomach and go down a scooter board ramp (a low-grade ramp made just for use with scooters—you could make one yourself if you don't own one). Holding an exercise wheel (a wheel with two handholds sticking out the sides) with both arms extended can help with focusing on the target and improving strength in the big postural muscles of the back and arms. Stack soft blocks as a target to knock down at the bottom of the ramp, or think of all the variations on a theme that this suggests, like:

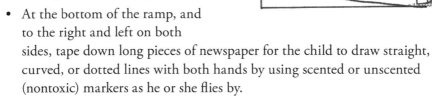

- Place the blocks at midline, then try building a tower to the right or to the left.

- Without using the wheel to steer, pick up puzzle pieces, small stuffed animals, or letters while rolling down the ramp.

- At the bottom of the ramp, and to the right and left on both sides, tape down long pieces of newspaper for the child to draw straight, curved, or dotted lines with both hands by using scented or unscented (nontoxic) markers as he or she flies by.

Human Spinner Game C

This activity <u>must be</u> customized for each child, who should be monitored closely by an occupational or vision therapist.

Before you start, be sure that the child will not be adversely affected by spinning. You will need a large rotating board, such as a lazy Susan, a rotating board used for plants to orient them to the sunlight, or a nystagmus board (used for evaluating the duration of eye movement after spinning in sensory processing tests). Have the child sit on the board or lie on it in a prone position; she will point with extended arms and feet as the board turns.

Arrange pieces of paper around the board, with instructions for various activities printed on them. The activities should be fun and new and provide just the right level of challenge for the child. Include an element of fun and novelty in the activities—for example, directions might include:

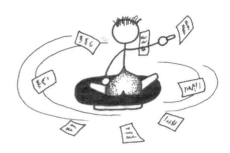

- Jump on the trampoline 10 times.
- Put the little finger of your right hand in your left ear.
- Count backward from 20 to one, skipping the numbers 13 and four.

A series of three activities per piece of paper is recommended, which should be graded from gross-motor activities to more fine-motor or cognitive ones. There may be six to 10 pieces of paper, perhaps with numbers on one side and corresponding directions to follow on the other side.

With the child on the rotating board, spin the child one turn and as the board slows down, have her point with an arm, leg, nose, elbow, or foot, while lying prone or sitting. Stop the spinning and have the child read and follow the directions on whichever piece of paper she is pointing to when she stops. Then do it all over again!

Bounce, Move, and Draw to the Music   C

Tape large sheets of paper to the wall. The child draws on the paper with nontoxic markers while bouncing or swaying to music. He may stand on a small trampoline or sit on a barrel or therapy ball. It's fun to draw and move to a march, a waltz, or an African, Native American, or Celtic rhythmic piece. Use whatever rhythm or mood helps the child. Be sure to give the child the necessary support if he is sitting on a barrel or a therapy ball!

One-Rope Saucer Swing   C

This activity requires a "saucer swing" on a rope, which is tied to a strong tree branch. Use a sturdy rope that is securely knotted around the tree limb! For beginners or younger children, an ordinary swing suspended with two ropes is less challenging. A rectangular or square (home-built) platform is often easier to balance on than the commercially available round, plastic saucer swings.

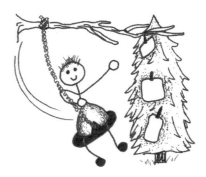

If there is a bush nearby, have the child swing over to reach it and try to touch higher and higher branches each time. Clothespins may be used to attach objects to a bush or to lower-hanging tree limbs, depending on the type of tree the saucer swing is hanging from. Old mismatched socks or small stuffed animals could be used as targets to reach for. As the child swings, have him try to grab objects placed in the bush or tree by using his hand(s) or feet.

Two-Rope Swinging   C

An ordinary two-rope swing can be used for a variety of games.

- Have the child sing with the rhythm of swinging; he can sing about what he sees as he swings or about how it feels to swing.
- The child can swing diagonally (with help from a grown-up) to reach for and strum a small harp, to hit a drum, or to reach for another object being held to the side of the swing.

Eye-Body and Eye-Hand Coordination Activities

"Zoom Ball" 🏠 Ⓔ 🌱 A C

This football-shaped ball, with ropes strung through it and handles at either end, can be played with by two people and is available at *sales@pressman-toy.com*.

This activity requires a lot of space, so it is better played outdoors on in a large room. To make the ball zoom back and forth across the ropes, the player holds onto the ropes and quickly extends his arms out to the side to make the ball zip over to the other player, and then quickly moves his hands together as the ball zooms back to him. This exercise is good for visual motor development, as well as for eye aiming.

Fish for Magnet Letters or Shapes Ⓔ C

Use a magnetic fishing pole. Adjust the length of the pole and line for the child's skill level—the longer the pole and line, the harder the fishing. Have the child fish from a platform swing or while sitting on a therapy ball or in a netted hammock or while sitting or standing in a suspended barrel at the therapy facility. The barrel can be securely placed on a platform swing or supported in a hammock, with the child climbing inside the barrel or sitting on top of it. The child can fish for objects placed on the floor or suspended from the ceiling with string. There are now some commercial puzzles made this way that could be used by a child who is sitting or standing, but sitting or standing alone lessens the visual-motor demand considerably.

Catching a Duck or Chicken Ⓔ ⌇ A C

This game can only be played on a farm and with supervision, so that the child and the fowl are safe. This game requires patience, calculation, judgment, stealth, and an understanding of critters! It also requires well-loved ducks and/or chickens. (Hint: "Polish" chickens, with feathers hanging down in their eyes, are easier to catch.) With adult supervision, allow the child to chase and try to catch a feathery friend. The calmer and more focused a child is, the more apt he is to be able to catch and hold one. This experience with the chickens builds empathy and knowledge of others' emotions and reactions. Try it and see.

Shaving Cream Games Ⓔ ⌇ A C

Many variations are possible with this game. Provide piles of towels and unscented, hypoallergenic shaving cream. Spread the cream over a large, smooth, washable, and secure surface, such as a tarp or large mats, and get ready to have some fun!

Here are a few activities children have participated in creating:

- In a suspended barrel, the child lies on his stomach and swoops over the shaving cream, creating designs with his hands or with scrubbers.
- Holding onto a trapeze, the child draws designs with his feet. One child playing this game drew the planets of the solar system with his toes, then slid from one to the other while giving the therapist a lesson about space.
- Some children actually like to roll around in the shaving cream!

The vestibular and deep tactile experience of this game, including the vigorous cleanup afterwards, prepares the child for more visually focusing activities and can be done just prior to drawing in the shaving cream. Be sure to wash all the soapy stuff off when the game is over so there's no itchiness from drying shaving cream on anyone's skin!

The Feely Game 🏠 🔍 🍎 A C

Have the child find objects that have been buried in a large container of dry rice, beans, lentils, or small pieces of pasta. To make the game easier and less tactilely challenging, simply place the objects in a sack or box. In terms of complexity, the progression of difficulty might be as follows:

- Have the child match objects from the container to sample objects positioned nearby.

- Once she's retrieved an object, have her match it to a picture of that object.

- Have her describe objects as she feels them, before she's brought them out to look at.

Finding Things in the Dark 🏠 🔍 C (Developing Visual Memory)

The first time you play this game, play with your eyes open. After that, play with your eyes closed. You can use actual objects at first, and then use pictures. The idea is to have the child place objects or pictures on a poster board or wall with Velcro, memorize where each object or picture is and feel where they are, and then close his eyes and try to "find them in the dark." The child should be stationary, perhaps standing on a gently sloped balance board.

Magnet Games 🏠 🔍 🍎 C

Using magnets above or below a tray, the child moves objects around on trails. This type of game can be made easily by using a flat piece of heavy cardboard or opaque plexiglass. Place small magnets of different sizes and shapes on top of the board and use the attracting magnet underneath to move the top magnets around a trail of your own design. Magnets and magnet games of this sort, such as Turtle Magnetic Marble Maze, are available in toy stores and therapy catalogs. You can begin using the commercial game by moving the magnets around from the top, as expected, and move on to a more kinesthetically challenging game by moving the magnet pieces from underneath the board. Magnet play can help the child build an increased awareness of visual motor–kinesthetic connections.

Rock, Throw, and Catch 🏠 Ⓔ A C

While standing on a rocker board, bouncing on a therapy ball, or sitting on a Move 'n' Sit inflatable cushion, the player moves, throws, and catches objects in time to music. Use up-tempo music with a straightforward beat, but not too fast. Throw soft pillows, stuffed animals, Koosh balls, and the like.

Scarves, Feathers, 🏠 Ⓔ 🍎 🌱 A C
and Streamers

Have the player march, twirl, or dance in time to music, using colored scarves and streamers. Drop a scarf, streamer, or feather from above the child's head and have her catch it as it drops down.

Koosh Ball Catch 🏠 Ⓔ 🍎 A C

Did you know that if you lie on your back and throw a Koosh ball straight up, you can play catch by yourself? Placing a picture or unbreakable mirror on the ceiling as a target directly above you helps make it easier and more fun! Koosh balls are soft, easily caught, and come in many colors and designs.

Irrigation Ditch or Stream 🌱 C
and Bridge Games

The following activity must have attentive, responsible adult supervision, especially for young children. The narrow, slow-moving, and not-too-deep irrigation streams of an organic farm in Colorado were ideal for the invention of these games.

- Float hoops or sticks from one bridge to another. The children scoop them up as they float by.
- Poohsticks (invented by Christopher Robin's friend, Winnie the Pooh): Throw sticks into the water from one side of the bridge, then run across to lie on your stomach to watch the sticks as they float by or to retrieve them from the other side of the bridge.
- Judge how to get into a rubber raft, how to steer, and how to get out without tipping the raft over. It's a challenge!

Croquet 🏠 Ⓔ 🌿 A C

This game, popular in Alice's Wonderland, requires a different kind of eye-hand coordination than that used in activities in which the ball is airborne (see Apple Baseball). It requires midline orientation and an ability to aim the mallet at the ball to propel it toward a target, which may be a wicket, or someone else's ball. Croquet sets are available at toy and sporting goods stores. This game definitely must be played outside.

Apple Baseball 🌿

A baseball bat and rotten apples make a hilarious game—be sure and wear old clothes! The novelty of this game strongly engages a child's interest (and tolerance of being messy, whether they are pitcher or hitter). It requires asymmetrical weight shifting and the ability to sight the ball and gauge the speed, orientation, and rotation at which the apple will arrive so that it can be hit. The child should hold the bat with both hands—the therapist may need to help them with their stance and remind them to keep their eye on the apple and not to laugh too hard.

Figure-Ground Activities

These activities develop what we call "figure-ground"—the ability to isolate one object and visually separate it from other background objects. These activities require that the child search for, identify, and find a particular object with a distinctive shape amidst a competing background.

Finding Four- (or Three-) Leaf Clovers in the Grass

The child needs to look through an array of green groundcover and be able to find a clover, as distinguished from grass or bindweed or another plant.

Picking Dandelion Greens

Have the child gather dandelions for a pet (such as a rabbit) to munch or for a salad. (Only do this if the dandelions have not been sprayed with herbicides.)

Finding Pictures and Shapes in the Clouds

Describe what you see in the clouds—can you see what someone else can?

"Wind"-Power Games 🏠 Ⓔ A C

Have the player use a straw or a length of flexible tubing to blow light objects toward a target—for example, blow little boats across a "lake" (you could use a bowl, bucket, or tub full of water) or blow cotton balls to a hit a target across a table.

Toy Basketball Blowing Pipe 🏠 Ⓔ 🍎 A C

These "Magic Blow Pipe" toys are available from *www.playworks.net/oral-motor-toys.html*. You can extend the stem of the pipe by attaching the length of flexible tubing you desire. Have the player bring the pipe closer or move it farther from his face while trying to get the little plastic ball into the basket. This requires the ability to aim the eyes together (converge) at near distances; extending the pipe allows the eyes to converge less, or diverge, while watching the ball stay balanced by using your breath.

Blowing Soap Bubbles Ⓔ 🍎 🌿 C

Have the child blow bubbles (or you can blow the bubbles for younger children), then have her pop them with her fingers as they float through the air.

Other Senses and Visual Attention

Sucking on Sour Candies, 🏠 🔍 🍎 🌱 A C
Pickles, or Lemon Pieces

Sour tastes help bring facial muscles and eyes into a more focused (aimed inward) state, called *convergence*. Sucking helps to bring facial muscles, including eye muscles, into a convergent posture. (Try it yourself and see!) After sucking on a sour food or piece of candy, encourage the child to attempt a near-vision task that was difficult for him previously, and see what happens!

Eye Movement Activities

Eye movement activities are important for living life. They are particularly critical for school achievement and sports skills. They allow the eyes to guide the body.

Wide Eye Stretches 🏠 Ⓔ 🍎 🌿 A C

This activity encourages the child to learn to look in all directions. It is hoped that the child can learn to do this activity with her head still, with eye movements separated from head movements. If this is not easy, start with head and eye movement together. Recite the following rhyme, and have the child do as you do. You could even turn it into a song!

> *Breathe in, look straight ahead—*
> > *Breathe out, look to the top of your head*
> *Breathe in, look straight ahead—*
> > *Breathe out, look to your right ear*
> *Breathe in, look straight ahead—*
> > *Breathe out, look to your left ear*
> *Breathe in, look straight ahead—*
> > *Breathe out, look down to your chin*
> *Breathe in, look straight ahead—*
> > *Breathe out, look down to your right*
> *Breathe in, look straight ahead—*
> > *Breathe out, look down to your left*
> *Breathe in, look straight ahead—*
> > *Breathe out, look up to your right*
> *Breathe in, look straight ahead—*
> > *Breathe out, look up to your left*
> *NOW, JUST BREATHE!*

It is always more fun to do exercises if imagination and stories are part of the game, especially when working with children. Two suggestions to make this activity more fanciful and interesting are:

- The story of the wandering spider—As the child's eyes move in various directions, he imagines that he is watching Charlotte, the friendly spider, spin her web. *Charlotte's Web,* by E. B. White, is a much-loved story about Wilbur ("some pig") and his friend, Charlotte the spider, which has now been made into a popular movie.

- The story of the strange clock is another example of how you can use your imagination to create a game. No props are needed for this activity. Imagine a clock with only eight numbers. By using his eyes, can the player find all the places on the clock where the numbers would be?

Wide Eye Pursuits 🏠 Ⓔ 🍎 🌿 A C

In this game, the eyes follow a smoothly moving target, such as a pen or a small flashlight. Move the target in figure eights, circles, and diagonal patterns.

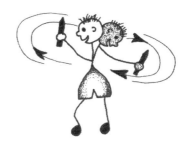

Again, stories can make this exercise more fun for children, and for adults, as well! It can also be helpful if noises that match the eye movements and the story can be incorporated into the exercise. Sounds can be created to mimic the movement of the characters—for instance, as the puppet or flashlight goes upward, the tone can get higher, and when the movement turns downward, the tone can go lower. Here are some ideas:

- Follow the movements of a finger puppet going side to side, up and down, and in a circle, doing figure eights and moving diagonally.

- Imagine that a fairy is trying out her new wings and that you are watching her loop around in all directions, side to side and up and down.

- Imagine that a new airplane is in the air for its very first trial flight and that you are the inventor who wants to be sure that it flies as it should. You can try "watching" the plane from the ground or pretend you're in the cockpit looking around you to see how your eye movements differ.

- An amazing new spaceship is on its first voyage, exploring every bit of outer space. You are watching it from space control headquarters, checking out every move of the spaceship. Remember to try to keep your head still, but move your eyes as if they are a searchlight. Can you describe what you are seeing as your eyes move around, or do you need to stop moving your eyes while you speak?

Two-Pen Jump 🏠 Ⓔ 🍎 🌱 A C

The first of these two activities requires two differently colored pens, perhaps one red and one blue. These exercises are important in developing ease of reading. They facilitate switching fixation quickly, zipping from one spot to the next.

Intervals between the fast-fixation movements and aiming the eyes should be varied. It is best to make the movements irregularly to add an element of surprise.

- Dueling pens—Call out the color of one pen, to draw the eyes to it. Then move the other pen, and draw the eyes to the new pen. Have the player look at the tip of the red or blue pen and fixate on it with her eyes. Then call out a pen color again, and so on.
- The "I spy" game—Use other small objects instead of pens. Move them around, keeping track of them out of the corner of your eye to be ready to look right at them when instructed. (Don't look until the very last second, and then look right at the person or object you want to catch with your eyes.)

Watch the Ball 🏠 Ⓔ C

The child rolls a ball or small toy car through tubes or barrels of varying sizes and lengths, straight ahead or from side to side. These can be left over from wrapping paper, aluminum foil, waxed paper, paper towels, or—to make the game easy— from small toilet-paper tubes. The tubes or barrels might have "windows" cut in them to enable the child to see the toy as it flies by. For a child who is distracted by everything around him or her, this game gives a clear visual aim. It can also be a way to encourage cooperative "give and take" play, where one child rolls the ball or marble through the tube to the therapist or another child, then has it rolled back to him or her, watching both sequences. It can also be played with a larger tube, such as a barrel, with a larger ball. This is a more basic game, involving more gross- than fine-motor skills.

Suspended-Ball Activities

These activities encourage visual-motor integration. The body reflects the movements of the eyes as the eyes follow the movements of the suspended ball.

Angels in the Snow   A C

If you have lived where there is snow in the winter, you know all about making snow angels. Lying down on your back and swishing your arms and legs to create an angel with wings and a long full skirt is sure to get snow down your neck and in your boots, but it's worth it! You can do these indoors or out.

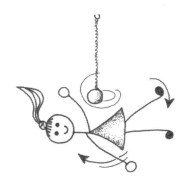

For this snow-angel exercise, use a soft, 3½-inch ball, suspended 3 feet from the floor. General instructions: First, have the child allow her eyes to move from side to side to watch the moving ball. Gradually, her arms and legs join in the game. When the ball is at midline, have her keep her arms and legs straight; when the ball moves to the right, have her move the right arm or leg to match the movement of the ball. Do the same with the left side of the body, as the ball swings toward the left.

- Lie on the floor underneath the ball, watching it as it swings. Your eyes should follow the ball in smooth movements. (The eyes need to follow the ball exactly, not using jerky movements or trying to anticipate what it will do.)

- Next, as your eyes follow the ball, move one arm at a time in rhythm with the ball; the right arm when the ball goes to the right, then the left arm as the ball swings to the left. (The arm should come out from beside the body out to the side, then up to the top of the head, returning to the side of the body when the ball is at midline).

- Add leg movements in tandem with the ball movements. (Again, when the ball is at midline, the legs are straight and together. Then, one or both legs move out to the appropriate side when the ball moves in that direction.)
- You can make this exercise more difficult by using eyes, arms, and legs together, instead of moving each individually. It may be difficult to coordinate the arms and legs, and one side of the body may want to "lead"—however, try to keep them in sync.

Another variation of this game is to have the child move only the right arm and leg, or the left, or the right arm and left leg together, and so on. This requires good coordination and the ability to initiate and suppress movement at will.

Ball in Wire 🏠 ⓔ A C

Suspend a soft ball from the ceiling, hanging slightly below waist height. Next, make a simple hoop from a wire coat hanger. (Start with a large wire hoop and larger ball.) Stand beside the ball in a relaxed, stable posture, and hold the hoop to keep the ball inside it without allowing the ball to touch the wire.

- Graduate to smaller balls and hoops to increase the level of difficulty.
- Vary the game by using different kinds and sizes of balls, and pretend they're planets moving in their orbits.
- "Capture" the ball by moving the wire up and down the string.
- Move in time to your favorite music, moving the hoop without disturbing the ball.
- Use Koosh balls, stuffed animals of different sizes, or a "planet" or "Earth ball."

Switch Hitting 🏠 Ⓔ A C

In this game, the player hits a suspended ball alternately with the right and left hand and says "right hand" or "left hand" with each hit.

- Use word opposites while hitting the ball with alternate hands.
  Examples might be hot-cold, sweet-sour, happy-grumpy, silly-serious, and north-south.

- Cover each hand with items that will provide different textures, such as oven mitts, shaving cream, or gloves.

Bunt Ball 🏠 Ⓔ A C

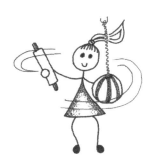

The player stands directly in front of a suspended ball and holds a dowel or rolling pin with both hands, one on each end, placed 6 inches away from the ball on each side. The player hits the ball back and forth between his hands, accurately and rhythmically. Vary where he connects with the ball: in the center, to the left of center, to the right of center, or in specific patterns. To facilitate this, tape of different colors can be applied to the dowel or rolling pin, such as blue in the very center, red on the right, and green on the left.

- Stand on a trampoline, a balance board, or a thick, soft mat while playing Bunt Ball.

- Count, recite the alphabet, or repeat nursery rhymes while playing.

- Move to some music, or even sing or hum while playing.

- Hit the ball while chanting jump-rope rhymes.

Chalkboard or Whiteboard Activity

This activity refines visual-motor integration.

Bimanual Board Circles

With a piece of chalk or marker in each hand, the player draws an X in the center of the chalkboard or whiteboard, directly in front of his nose. Then, backing up to a comfortable distance to use his hands, the player focuses on the X with both eyes while he begins to use both hands to draw circles. The head is kept still, and the child stands at a comfortable distance from the chalkboard or whiteboard while drawing.

- Start by reaching up to draw circles above the head.
- Then draw in toward the body, to midline.
- Then draw away from midline, to the sides of the body.
- Draw to the right using both hands.
- Draw to the left using both hands.

Variations include:

- Draw to the rhythm of a metronome, drum, or music with an easy, steady beat.
- Step away from the chalkboard and turn the circles into pictures to make the work "come alive." You could draw an animal, a home, a pie, a cake, a watermelon, a lake, a Ferris wheel, a merry-go-round, or a planet!
- Use templates to enhance the sensation of different shapes as they are being drawn. (A template is a sturdy piece of cardboard with a shape cut out that can be used to guide drawing with chalk on a board or pen on paper.)

- As you follow along the template with a pen or piece of chalk, pretend to be following a map and tell a story about the journey.
- Retell the story without using the template.
- Use different colors of chalk or ink in the right and left hands.
- Use chalkboards and whiteboards—there are different textures or "feels" to each of them.

Kirschner Arrow Chart

Call out the directions of the arrows in this chart, so that the player can move his eyes in the directions you name. If he likes, he can also call out each direction as he moves his eyes. You can say "right, left, up, down," or "12 o'clock, 3 o'clock, 6 o'clock, 9 o'clock," or even "north, south, east, west."

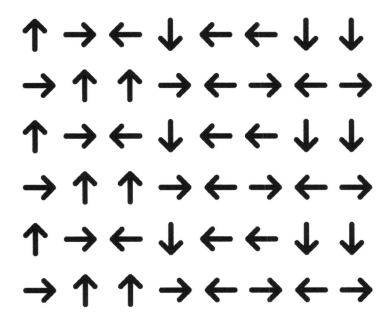

Variations include:

- Have the player jump forward, back, right, and left as the directions are called out.
- Have the player move his arms and legs in the direction of each arrow as it is called out.
- Add music or a rhythmic beat to the movements.

Visualization Activities

Visualization—the formation of mental visual images—is considered the crown jewel of vision ability. With imagery, it is possible to manipulate, move, change, and expand within "the mind's eye" to develop new perspectives and creativity. Visualization allows your mind to go beyond the here and now. It has no boundaries. Visualization is extremely important for academics and sports—you have to be able to "see" and manipulate ideas, numbers, and pictures "inside your head" to be truly proficient in these areas. There are unlimited possibilities with visualization activities. You can imagine or visualize with your eyes open or closed, while looking upward or straight ahead.

According to the occupational therapy literature, movement is important for providing the experience that is essential for visualization. Computers, TV, and simulators don't allow the muscles to experience a depicted activity. If they did, the Denver Broncos would not have to practice between games. The team members would only have to show up before the game and look at the play diagrams before taking the field. Instead, each member must proceed through the necessary stages of learning the skills required for a task or set of tasks. In the case of football:

- The body learns the patterns of movement associated with the game—the skills the body must be able to execute to play football.

- The visual system discriminates between similarities and differences—for instance, the Xs and Os mapped out on the coach's diagrams.

- As the play is practiced, the brain unites the information from the body (the physical skills used to play football) and visual system (play diagrams) until the movements become automatic.

Picture-on-the-Back Game   C

The child (or a group of children) chooses a category, and the adult thinks of a word in that category. For example, if the category is "weather," you might choose the word "blizzard." Using your index finger, "spell" the word, one letter at a time, on the child's back. Record each letter on paper or a blackboard (or see below) when the child guesses it. You can either spell things correctly, or scramble the order of the letters. Once all the letters have been "spelled" and recorded, the child or the group can unscramble the letters and guess the word.

For alternate modes of spelling (not on the back):

- Use unscented, hypoallergenic shaving cream on a large cookie sheet or other surface, and draw with the elbows or feet.

- Put each letter on a separate piece of paper so that they can be easily rearranged.

- Once the child has guessed the word, he can write the word with a vibrating pen (available in therapy catalogs) to reinforce the tactile experience while watching the letters (the visual aspect) emerge.

- Use pudding or applesauce to transform this game into a treat involving the visual, motor, olfactory, and taste systems! Have the child mix and shake instant pudding in a quart jar, jumping up and down, shaking diagonally or from side to side to mix the pudding. Then, spread the pudding on a cookie sheet or pizza pan. Let the child "draw" with his tongue on the "pudding palette"—try drawing pictures or letters. Drawing with the tongue gives a clear feeling of the shape of the letters.

Flashlight Tag   C

An adult sits with a flashlight on one side of a bedsheet or translucent divider. The child sits on the other side. As the adult traces patterns with the flashlight, the child follows along with her finger or with her own flashlight.

A large translucent barrel—the type used to store food products—is perfect for this activity, but you need to be lucky and resourceful to find one. The child must be small enough to fit comfortably inside the barrel—the adult uses the flashlight from the outside. Lois found hers at a ski boot–manufacturing facility.

Pictures in Your Mind 🏠 Ⓔ A C

A child needs to be able to visualize to allow him to shift his attention from the physical world of movement, touch, hearing, and sight to the symbolic world of letters, words, ideas, and imagination.

Appropriate visualization activities can be performed by children or adults by varying the complexity of the task to accommodate the needs and the age of the individual.

Have the player close his eyes. Begin this game by asking, "What do you see?" This works better than asking, "Can you see something?" Asking if a person can see something will often result in an automatic "No."

Then offer suggestions, and have the player tell you what he or she is visualizing. Here are some ideas:

- Imagine a light bulb. Can you make it warmer, brighter, or a different color?

- Imagine playing with parquetry blocks (blocks made of geometric shapes and patterns) or a geoboard (a grid of pegs laid out on a flat board), playing memory games, or finding hidden pictures.

- Imagine different colors, sounds, sizes, textures, tastes, temperatures, movements, speeds, smells, rhythms, and spaces. Imagine different levels of brightness and clearness.

- Imagine using different aspects of communication, such as humor or exaggeration.

- Imagine whistling and singing.

If encouraging and imaginative responses are flowing, try introducing a game such as "My Ape Is."

"My Ape Is"

This game encourages humor and imagination—the sillier the better! Participants take turns imagining an ape and describing how it looks. One player might say, "My ape wears polka-dotted socks." The next player adds, "My ape is purple and wears polka-dotted socks, and he just got a mosquito bite on his elbow." The next player might add, "Well, my ape is purple and wears polka-dotted socks and has a mosquito bite on his elbow, and he has enormous ears with six earrings on each."

This game could just as easily be changed to "My Cabbage Is" or "My Spaceship Is" or "My Alligator Is." There is no limit to the possibilities!

Handling Fears and Criticism

Visualization can be a way to handle fears and criticism. Close your eyes and remember being in an uncomfortable situation. Remember how you felt and what you said to yourself. Now stop the movie in your head and step out so that you see the picture, including yourself and the other person involved. Move the picture several feet away. Now, start the movie all over again, but before you do, imagine that you and the other person are meeting for the first time and are anxious to know each other better.

Inject humor or exaggeration, a sense of comfort or security, or differing levels of brightness into your memory. Use any technique you need to decrease the discomfort level and to increase your confidence and sense of comfort and the comfort level of the other person.

When you find yourself in a similar situation in the future, think about the humorous or friendly movie that you've created, with yourself in the picture looking confident and strong. This strategy allows you to use any important feedback you may get and also allows you to see the other person with more objectivity. Review these points the next time you find yourself in a challenging situation:

- Visualization can be a useful way to handle fears or criticism.
- Visualization can be a way to remember how a situation felt—the feelings, sounds, smells, ambient temperature, and the overall picture.
- It can help to imagine stepping out of the situation and seeing the picture from several feet away.

- Visualization allows the use of humor and exaggeration and the introduction of a sense of comfort and security. Anything about the situation can be changed to improve your memory of it.

Spelling Visualization

Spelling visualization can facilitate spelling comprehension. Use a colored marker to write a word on an index card or flash card. Hold the card up and away from the player's face. Have the person make a picture of the word in her mind and "snap a camera picture."

Take the card away and ask the person to describe the picture: Have her describe its color, size, texture, and brightness level. (Her eyes may be open or closed.) Have the person trace the letters of the word in the air with her finger or by using eye movements or an imaginary magic wand. Spell the word not by using the actual letter, but by indicating the height of the letter. For example, the "tall letters" include *b, d, f, h, k, l*, and *t*, and a sound for these letters could be "woop." The "long letters" include any letter that goes below the line, such as *g, j, p, q*, and *y*; their sound could be "la." The "short letters" include all the other letters of the alphabet, and their sound could be "ch." The word "cat" would be spelled "small, small, tall," or "ch, ch, woop." The word "elephant" would be "ch, woop, ch, la, woop, ch, ch, woop."

If the person still has difficulty seeing the entire word in her mind, break it into groups of three or four letters. Have her write the word as she sees it as a picture. Once the person sees the complete word as a picture, have her call out the letters backward. (This demonstrates that the word has truly been seen in the mind and that visualization is being used, not auditory recall. The smoothness and rapidity with which the child spells can also tell you that the word was truly visualized.) Then, try spelling the word forward while jumping forward and backward while jumping backward.

After developing the strategy, visualization can improve spelling and other memorization activities. When reading to a child, stopping and creating pictures on paper or in the mind helps the child retain more of the story and enhances the understanding of it. To facilitate this ability to truly see the word, it may be helpful to first look at an isolated picture of an elephant, then perhaps add the word elephant on top of the picture, and then finally, put it in context—that is, see it in a jungle setting. The more colorful, detailed, and layered the image is, the more it will be remembered.

Bouncing a Ball
to Learn Spelling

Parents can suggest movement patterns that will increase a child's skill level to reach the gestalt of learning. For example, a child who experiences difficulty with spelling is demonstrating an inability to visualize words.

Adding body movement patterns—such as dribbling a ball in the shape of the letters being used, or dribbling over a letter to spell a word—will speed up the learning process. You could draw the letters on the pavement with sidewalk chalk— or, indoors, draw letters on a large piece of paper. Movement of the body allows the entire activity of spelling to move to the subconscious in less time. As the child gains control over his body, he can devote more energy to learning to spell.

The following chart explains how to use a bouncing ball to spell words, with a general rule of spelling one letter per bounce. After a word is presented to the child, have the child spell the word forward (one letter per bounce), then backward (also one letter per bounce). Then, ask the child, "What letter comes before/after the letter..." Difficulty is outlined by grade level:

Grade Level	Ball Type	Ball-Bouncing Instructions (One Bounce per Letter)	Word Presentation
Kindergarten	Large play ball	Bounce and catch the ball with both hands.	Write the word on a large piece of paper.
1st Grade	Tennis ball	Bounce the ball with the right hand, catch it with the left hand. Bounce the ball with the left hand, catch it with the right hand.	Write the word on a large piece of paper.
2nd Grade	Tennis ball	Dribble the ball with alternating hands.	Have the child visualize the word.
3rd Grade	Tennis ball	Dribble the ball in a pattern. Dribble twice with the right hand, then once with the left hand. Switch.	Have the child visualize the word.
4th Grade	A ball 1½ inches in diameter	Dribble the ball in a pattern. Dribble three times with the left hand, then twice with the right hand. Switch.	Have the child visualize the word.
5th-6th Grade	1-inch super bouncer	Dribble in patterns of three. Dribble once on the right, twice on the left, three times on the right. Repeat. Switch.	Have the child visualize the word.
7th-8th Grade	1-inch super bouncer	Dribble in patterns of three, using only two fingers.	Have the child visualize the word.

Table adapted from *Fields of Vision—The Newsletter of Achievers Unlimited, Inc.* Used with permission. January 1998 issue, Vol 2, No 5. (This resource—Achievers Unlimited—is no longer available.)

Reading Comprehension

Mildred Odess Gifford, author of *The Power of Imagery*, describes how to help children develop better reading comprehension. Some of her strategies include the following:

- Have the student read a sentence, close his eyes, and visualize what he has just read, then open his eyes and read the sentence again.
- Have the student close her eyes while a word is spelled aloud several times, then ask her to imagine writing it on the chalkboard, tracing the imagined letters in her mind each time (not in the air).
- Have the student trace each letter of a word in the air as the word is spoken, then spell it aloud.

For a child who has difficulty with syllables, Ms Gifford uses the following strategy:

- Ask the child to close his eyes and visualize himself writing the problem syllables several times.
- Pronounce the first syllable and touch his left arm, saying, "on this side."
- Touch his chest for the middle syllable sound.
- Pronounce the last syllable, touching his right arm and saying, "on this side."
- Next, practice putting the sounds together, working from the mental images and touching left arm, chest, and right arm. (For example, to say "elephant," the child would say "el" while touching his left arm, "e" while touching his chest, and "phant" while touching his right arm.)
- Last, look at the printed syllables and read them aloud without spelling them first, encouraging the child to "feel" the sounds.

Creative Writing Visualization

If a child is having trouble with a writing assignment, break down the process into the following steps. Have the student visualize a story in her mind and use it to create a cartoon sequence. Add as many specific details as possible, like color, brightness, speed, and sound. If she wishes, have her draw pictures and put the cartoon strip in motion to see it as a movie. Now, have her write the story as she visualized it, without emphasizing spelling, grammar, or neatness until the story is complete. Then have her edit the story.

Share these tips to make writing more fun:

- Write easily and softly.
- Use large writing utensils or a pencil grip.
- When making the pictures, paint from the shoulder.
- Use a keyboard or computer to reduce the frustration of editing and recopying by hand.
- Visualize successful completion of the task.
- If the child gets stuck in creating the story, gently remind her to review the movie and write from her pictures. Fear and self-criticism create writing blocks.

- If she is overwhelmed with ideas, try having her make a picture outline with differently colored markers.
- Try tape-recording a story, then having her listen to the tape and build her picture. Then she can write it.
- Have fun!

Remember and Follow Directions

If remembering and following directions is a problem, use the following visualization method:

- Give instructions to the child.
- Direct the child to look up and visualize himself carrying out the requested directions.
- Have the child make a moving picture of it in his mind, then rerun the picture if there is confusion.

Here's an example: Picture yourself walking into your bedroom, opening your closet, taking out a pair of shoes, and putting them on. Now review your moving picture in your mind, and then carry out each step you visualized.

Performance Visualization

Visualizing an upcoming musical or athletic performance can be a very helpful method for reducing anxiety and preparing for the event. To enhance your performance—whether it be music, dancing, singing, athletics, or acting—try these ideas:

- Imagine yourself performing.
- See and feel yourself in the actual performance, as well as imagining yourself as a bystander watching the performance.
- See the entire process with as many details as you can, including movement, touch, sound, smell, and temperature.
- See the performance from different angles.
- Change the speed of your mental "movie."
- Break down your mental pictures by category: preparation, actual performance, completion, winding down, and returning back to present reality.

- See if you can conjure up the physical feeling of what it's like to have a good performance experience. What does it feel like to perform well?

For a complete, detailed book on using visualization, see the newly published (in 2010) *See It. Say it. Do it! The Parent's & Teacher's Action Guide to Creating Successful Students and Confident Kids,* by Dr Lynn F. Hellerstein.

Computers and Vision

Do you spend time on a computer? Many people do, both children and adults. We all know that computers can be visually stressful. Here are a few fun ideas to help you cut down on visual stress when you work on a computer.

- Make sure that you are seated directly in front of your computer and looking at it straight on.

- Sit with your feet flat on the floor and your knees and hips at a 90° angle, with your back straight. You might try sitting on an exercise or therapy ball instead of a chair, or experiment with the very best sitting arrangement (ergonomically) for your body.

- Try to position your monitor slightly below your line of sight and 20 to 26 inches away from you.

If your computer setup will allow it, and you frequently copy information from a book or page, vary the side of the computer on which you place the book or pages. Copy information while looking to the right on Mondays, Wednesdays and Fridays, switch it over to the left on Tuesday and Thursdays, then reverse the days the following week.

- Eliminate glare from your screen by turning it away from any windows.

- Place colors around you that relax you and remind you to be present in the world and not just involved with the information on the computer.

- Place soft fabrics, textures, and drapes behind your monitor that will help you "ground" when you pause in your work.

- Have a picture or photo, painting, or poster nearby that has some depth to it. Pause from looking at your screen occasionally and gaze into the picture to relax your focus.

- Remember to take visual breaks from your work. You can look at your drapes, at a picture, or out the window—or just daydream. Get up and walk around every half-hour or so. You can continue to think about your work if you wish, but get your body moving and remember to relax your visual focus.

- Sound may help you—experiment with listening to enjoyable soft music, played on your computer, if possible.

- Some people find that looking at a computer screen is very stressful. There are special spectacle lens prescriptions that can alleviate this by using the properly prescribed lens power and/or tinting and glare coatings. It may also be possible to get contact lenses with a computer prescription. A full visual evaluation is recommended, however, with emphasis on the distance of the computer from your eyes—be sure to bring all the specifications about your computer setup with you.

- Remember: Computers and keyboards are only tools. They should make your work easier—try to think of it as your friend and colleague instead of a taskmaster. (This idea was the brainchild of the late behavioral optometrist Elliott Forrest, author of *Stress and Vision,* who recognized that those who use the keyboard as a friend have much less visual stress than those who feel it is a taskmaster).

- There are commercial teas and herbs available to refresh and soothe tired eyes. Consult with a naturopath or an herbalist for specific recommendations.

If you work indoors most of the time, under artificial lighting, please be sure to spend time in natural light every day, either outdoors or with candles or firelight at night. Full-spectrum lighting can be important in making your workday at the computer healthier for your eyes.

Is Sooner Always Better?

Rebecca E. Hutchins, OD, FCOVD

In this new millennium, the pace of life has truly accelerated. Families are busy, children's lives are scheduled with all kinds of activities, and childhood seems to have been condensed almost out of existence. One place this is clearly evident is in formal schooling and organized learning. In the 1950s and 60s, relatively few children attended nursery school (as it was then called), and some did not even attend kindergarten. First grade was usually the initial contact with formal education. This was the child's first experience with reading, writing, and arithmetic. Now, many children attend preschool, and there seems to be a demand for children to master certain skills at earlier ages and in lower grades.

Rudolpf Steiner created the Waldorf Schools in the early 1920s.[1] He designed the elementary-school curriculum to be developmentally appropriate. Waldorf students practice manual skills, such as hammering or knitting, as preparation for writing in kindergarten. Writing the alphabet is initially performed by using pictures and by telling an ongoing story about each letter. These skills are practiced by doing artwork in special booklets. Reading is not taught until the child is ready and does not usually occur until the 3rd grade. Prior to that time, children are encouraged to vicariously experience the written word by listening to storytellers. The stories are read aloud, and the children create and perform puppet shows to tell the stories.

In the 1930s, Arnold Gesell, MD, designed a comprehensive research project with which to observe human development, beginning in infancy and following the same individuals through childhood.[2] He stressed that not all children develop at the same rate. Boys tend to develop some skills at a later time than girls. Overall, he advised parents to wait until a child was developmentally ready before encouraging mastery of learning-related skills, even if this meant holding a child back a year in school.

Howard Gardner has written several books since the mid-1980s, describing types of intelligence.[3-4] He proposed that a child may be highly skilled in some areas and yet perform quite poorly in others. His goal was, and continues to be, to encourage schools to teach lessons designed to accommodate a child's learning styles, allowing the student to absorb knowledge in his most accessible mode. Gardner noted:

> There is now copious evidence to suggest that developmental domains are…independent of one another, with advances in one area often failing to signal comparable advance in other areas. Thus for example, a child's first meaningful utterances occur well before the first meaningful drawings. Unlike the carefully interlocking parts of a watch, the structures of the mind and of the brain seem to be able to evolve in different directions and at different paces.[3]

This acknowledgement underscores the fact that development in one area may precede that of another. This explains why a child may not be equally ready to learn all the subjects required of her in the classroom. At least a part of Gardner's solution to this dilemma is to present information in several different ways: through music and movement and construction tasks, not just by means of lecture or reading. Such a solution, however, does not address the more basic question of whether the material presented is developmentally appropriate.

Janet Healy wrote two books on brain development, primarily for the lay person.[5,6] I believe they both hold profound information. The first book, perhaps better known, is entitled, *Endangered Minds: Why Our Children Don't Think and What We Can Do about It.*[5] It is well worth reading for parents, as well as for optometrists. The second book, *Your Child's Growing Mind: A Practical Guide to Brain Development and Learning From Birth to Adolescence,*[6] has a chapter entitled, "If the Train Is Late, Will We Miss the Boat? Developmental Timetables and Learning to Pay Attention." The beginning of this chapter states: "One of the hardest things for everyone to understand is that bright children are not necessarily on the fastest train. Many problems of 'underachievement' result from an incongruity between the child's neurological pattern or timetable and the expectations of the family and school."[6]

When my son entered kindergarten in the 1997–1998 school year, he, his father, and I were all equally excited and expectant. All three of us soon became frustrated and overwhelmed with the skills expected—nay, demanded—of him and his classmates. We had exposed him to letters and numbers. We had let him play with workbooks and games about letter and number recognition but had not exposed him to the formal instruction of writing numbers and letters or of reading.

Our son brought home a picture he had drawn during the first week of school. In an unformed scrawl was written, "I stayed home all day." We asked him who wrote it, and he said he did, with the teacher's help. As the weeks passed, he was expected to write on most activities, both in his kindergarten class and during "enrichment classes," which occupied the afternoon hours. Our son had some sensory-integration and fine-motor-control problems, and, consequently, he found these demands frustrating. Soon, he was coming home complaining, "Everybody can read and write but me."

I began volunteering in his classroom once a week. I knew my son's skills were average to above average when compared with those of the other children in his class, but we couldn't convince him that he was not inferior. We solved the problem by moving him to a Waldorf-model "focus" public school, where these reading and writing skills aren't expected until later. He immediately became less anxious and more confident in all areas of school performance.

Clearly, our son was not yet ready to read and write. It's possible that, 30 years ago, these issues would not have been a problem. One of my 20-something staff members reminisced that the only letters and numbers she was exposed to in kindergarten were on Sesame Street videos. My husband, who was schooled in New Mexico, didn't start classes until 1st grade. However, I have seen children in my practice whose parents are concerned about their children's ability to enter a parochial-school kindergarten because they do not yet know all their numbers and letters. I have encountered parents who have had their kindergarten children tutored so they would be reading well enough to enter 1st grade!

I propose that kindergarten should be designed to help children understand social skills, communicate, and work with others in preparation for academics in 1st grade. Much of the work in my son's first school was developmentally inappropriate. In the teacher's defense, she had 26 children of varying abilities and interests, with no paraprofessional or aide to help her. The teacher assigned many paper-and-pencil tasks. These tasks were usually performed while sitting at a desk, and they were not easy or comfortable for many of the children, including my son. Of course, she may have been knowledgeable and have wanted to use more concrete teaching activities but couldn't, because of the size of the class. Healy, in *Your Child's Growing Mind,* suggests that parents "march on your local school district and demand to know why they are not following developmental guidelines in their classrooms."[6]

She adds later that, "Meanwhile, we must insist that teaching at every grade level remains suitable for the wide variety of developmental needs in the children it is meant to serve."[6]

It may also be true that schools are actually bowing to pressure from the parents who are requesting, sometimes demanding, academic instruction at younger and younger ages. I receive brochures that advertise programs to teach my infant to read. Why, I wondered, would I push reading on a 6-month-old baby? His visual skills are clearly not yet ready. Is the brain not programmed to unfold in a certain pattern and at an appropriate rate? As a behavioral optometrist, I am amazed at the spectrum of visual skills I see, especially in the preschool and early school-aged population. I once believed that I could predict a child's reading ability by assessing his or her ocular motor skills during pursuits or saccades. However, when I began receiving referrals of gifted children, I would see preschool-level tracking in a child whose parent assured me he read at a 6th- or 8th-grade level. Even so, when these children did the remedial work necessary to improve their eye movements, there were improvements in many areas. I had a theory at the time that most of these children, who began to read at 2 to 5 years of age, did not yet possess the visual control necessary for smooth, efficient eye movements. Since they were motivated to succeed in reading and were in the gifted range, they had not been required or allowed to learn adequate ocular-motor skills. These gifted children with poor eye movements appeared to be masters at gleaning subject matter in spite of poor eye movements.

Examples

I recently examined a 2nd grader. The child was exhibiting problems in reading, and, in fact, I believed that his eye-movement skills were comparable to a normally developing 3-year-old. The father asked about not pursuing vision therapy but rather waiting for the child to mature. He asked if it was reasonable to assume that development would take care of the problem. The mother countered that she sits down to read each night with the child and that he is incredibly frustrated when faced with the written word. My recommendation was vision therapy for this child to help his skills improve to an age-appropriate level. As the child's ocular-motor skills improved, an improvement in his schoolwork was observed, as well as a decrease in his stress level as related to school.

Another child, a 5-year-old, demonstrated borderline-average vision skills for his age but was placed in an accelerated 1st grade because he tested as gifted. I believed he would benefit from being placed in a traditional kindergarten program and that, by the next year, his visual system might be ready for the demands of 1st grade. The parents agreed, and the next year, the child performed well in the accelerated 1st grade.

The Optometric Role

Optometrists can play a pivotal role in advising parents, when it comes to a child's placement in school. A solution to placement in an academic curriculum is to follow the concept of developmental readiness and how child readiness applies directly to formal schooling. A minimal level of developmental maturity should be assured. Many children are not developmentally ready for formal schooling until age 6½ or 7.[7] A proper maturational level for academic participation will better ensure the child's readiness for school achievement. The child should be evaluated by developmental specialists, and agreement should be arrived upon by professionals in the fields of both child development and education.

I propose that the role of the optometrist is to propose and provide answers to the following questions:

A. What visual-motor and visual-information processing skills are necessary for children of a given age or grade level to succeed academically?
B. Is the individual child ready for these age/grade challenges?
C. How can optometrists help parents and teachers learn about developmental readiness?
D. How can we convince educational professionals and society that "sooner is NOT always better"?
E. How can we allow children to develop more at their own pace, without familial or societal guidelines affecting their self-esteem?

In summary, if we ask a child to learn a skill at a time when he or she is not developmentally ready, we risk frustrating the child. This can be damaging to the child's self-image and possibly derail the activities that the maturational internal clock has planned for this time period. At the risk of sounding simplistic, can't we let children be children, at least through kindergarten?

Optometric testing and assessments can prove useful in the evaluation of vision skills and visual perceptual/cognitive skills, on the basis of normative data. Children who are late bloomers are often labeled as "needing special help," when a therapeutic dose of time and patience might be all that is needed. The profession, particularly behavioral optometry, has a tradition of keeping abreast of the current knowledge about brain and/or vision development and learning capabilities. The behavioral optometrist should advise parents to either support remediation and/or delay formal academics, whichever is more appropriate.

A Waldorf curriculum[1] is not desirable or accessible to many families. The Gardner Multiple Intelligence model may allow some children to access knowledge in their preferred mode, and this method is currently being taught.[3,4] Still, neither of the programs addresses the basic question of developmental readiness. Gesell's solution of holding children back won't work in a system in which reading and writing skills are required in kindergarten.[2] Perhaps some of the burgeoning new research on brain development will become available to inform parents, teachers, and schools about the timing and the development of the visual system. The development of the total child—the visual, speech- and auditory-processing, sensory-integration, and motor skills—all apply to the training of young minds and bodies.

It is my belief that our fast-paced life and fast-food mentality must NOT influence our attitudes toward learning. We should not advocate academics at younger and younger ages. This shift may not only affect a child's self esteem but can create an "all work and very little play" mentality, which minimizes the fun and nonacademic learning of childhood. It is clear to me that "sooner is not always better," especially when it comes to learning.

References

1. Ogletree EJ, Ujlaki V. School Readiness and Rudolf Steiner's Theory of Learning. http://eric.ed.gov/ERICWebPortal/custom/portlets/recordsDetails/detailmini.jsp?_nfpb=true&_&ERICExtSearch_SearchValue_0=ED310841&ERICExtSearch_SearchType_0=no&accno=ED310841. Accessed December 12, 2008.

2. Gesell A, Ilg F, Bullis G. *Vision: Its Development in Infant and Child.* Santa Ana, CA: Optometric Extension Program Foundation, Inc; 1998.

3. Gardner H. *Frames of Mind: The Theory of Multiple Intelligences.* New York, NY: Basic Books; 1993.

4. Gardner H. *The Unschooled Mind: How Children Think and How Schools Should Teach.* New York, NY: Basic Books; 1991:28-29.

5. Healy J. *Endangered Minds: Why Our Children Don't Think and What We Can Do about It.* New York, NY: Touchstone Books; 1990.

6. Healy J. *Your Child's Growing Mind: A Guide to Learning and Brain Development from Birth to Adolescence.* Rev ed. Bantam Doubleday Dell Publishing Group; 1994:66, 71-72.

7. Rosner J. Reading readiness. In: Garzia R, ed. *Vision and Reading.* St Louis, MO: Mosby-Year Books, Inc; 1996:49.

This article is reprinted with permission of The Journal of Behavioral Optometry. It was originally published in 2009, Volume 20.

Losing Sleep?
Light May Be a Culprit!
Rebecca E. Hutchins, OD, FCOVD

We all learn as children how bears hibernate during the winter. How do they know when to do this? It is governed by the timing and intensity of light. Humans, too, are affected by so-called "circadian rhythms," which influence sleep-wake cycles, jet lag, attention and arousal, eating and drinking habits, and many aspects of metabolism.

Rods and cones are the photoreceptors we all learned about in school. In the beginning of the 21st century, a previously unknown photoreceptor, melanopsin, was discovered. This photoreceptor transmits information to the pineal gland and is instrumental in controlling the production of melatonin.

Melanopsin is triggered by light of a specific wavelength, which we perceive as blue (460–480 nm). Light, especially blue light, suppresses the production of melatonin, which thereby affects our ability to sleep (as melatonin contributes to the inducement of sleep).

So how does this affect us in our daily lives? It means that exposure to light during the night prevents the expected triggering of melatonin production. The types of light this might encompass include sunlight if you're trying to sleep during the day, a bright night-light in your bedroom, street lights or a neighbor's lights shining in your bedroom window, light enveloping an urban area that is never truly dark, a lamp used during the night to read, or light from your TV or computer.

In fact, many researchers in this field believe that we should go without blue light for at least 2 hours prior to sleep.

You may wonder about the primary sources of blue light in our environment. If you guessed computers and televisions, you're right! This means that watching TV or using the computer right before bed or during the night—or sleeping in a room with a TV or computer on—is actually detrimental to our ability to get a good night's sleep.

By evaluating night-shift workers, researchers found that amber-tinted lenses, or other tints that block the blue-light wavelengths, allow a person to work in light, yet produce melatonin as if in darkness. As Dr James Phelps, a psychiatrist from Corvallis, Oregon, puts it, "blue light is the light that counts," and blocking it can be one option.

If you have sleep issues and wonder if blue light might be related, you may want to consider some of the following options:

- Turn off the computer or television 2 hours prior to bedtime.
- Cover or hide light-emitting diode clocks and other devices.
- Keep the bedroom uniformly dark during the night—use light-blocking shades if there is outdoor light that comes in a window.
- If a night-light is needed, consider one that is rated as having a low blue-light level.
- When it is not possible to eliminate computer or television use 2 hours prior to bedtime, consider the use of tinted lenses that block the unwanted wavelengths.
- If using tinted lenses, choose a frame that blocks as much light from the side as possible.
- Work to minimize or eliminate "light at night" pollution in your area.

References

Bodfield R. Vision problems can be source of kids' bad grades. *Arizona Daily Start.* September 2, 2009.

Forrest E. *Stress and Vision.* Santa Ana, CA: Optometric Extension Program Foundation; 1988.

Furth H, Wachs H. *Thinking Goes To School: Piaget's Theory in Practice.* New York, NY: Oxford University Press; 1982.

Getman GN. *How To Develop Your Child's Intelligence.* Santa Ana, CA: Optometric Extension Program; 1993.

Gifford M. *Watch Learning Problems Disappear: The Power of Imagery.* GiffOdess Books; 1999.

Kavner R. *Your Child's Vision: A Parent's Guide To Seeing, Growing, and Developing.* New York, NY: Simon & Schuster; 1985.

Lyons EB. *How To Use Your Power of Visualization.* Red Bluff, CA: Lyons Visualization Series; 1980.

Nurek K, Wendelburg D. *Vision Development: 0-3, An Observe & Play Workbook.* Fond du Lac, WI: Achievers Unlimited; 1996.

Newsletter: *Begin Where They Are.* Fond du Lac, WI: Achievers Unlimited; 1996.

Seiderman A, Marcus S. *20/20 Is Not Enough: The New World of Vision.* New York, NY: Fawcett Crest; 1991.

Glossary

20/20 Acuity—The ability to see a certain-sized letter or picture from 20 feet away, which has been designated as having "normal" vision; the larger the denominator, the worse the acuity

Acuity—Clarity of sight; the ability to see objects clearly up close and at a distance

Amblyopia—Lazy eye; a healthy eye that cannot see clearly, even with the best prescription, which is caused by strabismus (one or both eyes turning inward or outward), pronounced astigmatism, or differences in refraction between the two eyes

Anticipate—To move the eyes in the direction one thinks an object will move, not really waiting to track the object itself

Astigmatism—A refractive error, where the eye is not spherical or round but football shaped and needs a cylindrical lens to provide good acuity

Behavioral model of vision—Dr A. M. Skeffington initiated the behavioral model of vision in the 1920s. Vision cannot be separated from the total individual or from any other sensory system, as it is integrated into all human performance. Vision is learned and therefore trainable. Many visual problems appear to be triggered by environmental factors, which may be developmental or stress induced. Many visual problems can be prevented or reduced by environmental modifications, like near-point lenses or vision therapy.

Directionality—The ability to orient to and visualize direction in space, whether it be right, left, up, or down, or when projected on paper or a map

Enhancement—The process of improving skills, whether or not a problem has been identified

Ergonomics—The study of posture and movement in creating the optimal positions while working (as at a desk) to prevent discomfort and damage to the joints

Eye crossing—A tendency for one or both eyes to turn in toward the nose

Eye aiming—The ability to aim both eyes at the same point in space; this is important so that the two eyes stimulate corresponding points in the visual cortex of the brain to produce a three-dimensional image

Eye drifting—A tendency for one eye to turn out, toward the ear

Eye movement—The ability to smoothly move the eyes to follow and to do accurate point-to-point movements

Eye teaming—The ability to aim or point both eyes together so that the brain can superimpose the resultant images for good depth perception

Figure ground—The ability to see one object and separate it from the background, as in finding a four-leaf clover in a field of clover

Fine-motor coordination—The ability to control small muscles of the body comfortably and efficiently, as in handwriting or tying a "fly" onto your fishing line or knitting with the fingers

Fixation saccades—Point-to-point eye movements, such as those used in reading words on a page

Focusing—The ability to see clearly at close range or change from near vision to distance vision and back

Gross-motor coordination—The ability to control the large muscles of the body comfortably and easily, such as when kicking or hitting a ball

Integration—The ability to put two skills together, such as vision and movement

Laterality—Knowing one's right side from the left side of the body

Lenses—Optical devices used to provide the eye with different visual experiences, such as making the eyes focus in or relax focus

Localize—The ability to tell where something is located in space and to turn the eyes, ears, nose, and body toward it

Motor planning (praxis)—The fluent integration and flow of thought and movement; purposeful movement is praxis in action

Nystagmus—Involuntary, rhythmical, repeated oscillations of one or both eyes

Physiological diplopia—The normal phenomenon of seeing two images in space at a distance closer to or beyond where the eyes are aimed; this is used to explore and train binocularity

Prisms—Optical devices that make an object appear at a different location or encourage the eyes to move up, down, right, or left

Progressive overload—Beginning with a simple activity, then adding components to keep it interesting and raise the level of difficulty—for instance, hitting a ball, then hitting it rhythmically, then saying a letter of the alphabet each time the ball is hit

Proprioception—The awareness of ourselves that is gained through muscles and joints and through other receptors with our bodies (in Latin, *proprio* means "within," and *incipere* means "to take up" or "to begin")

Pursuits tracking—Smooth eye movements, as in following a moving object

Refraction—The clinical examination of the eye to determine the need for glasses; involves the use of a large piece of equipment placed in front of the eyes, called a *phoroptor* or *refractor*

Saccades—Point-to-point eye movements, such as those used in jumping from word to word when reading

Sensory integration—The process of taking in information about the world around us with all of our senses and from inside our own bodies; through integrating and organizing the senses of vision, touch, movement, muscle sense, hearing, and smell, we are able to interact comfortably and efficiently in work and play

Sequencing—The ability to do things in a certain order

Spatial orientation—The ability to see how things relate in space, such as the difference between the letters "b" and "d," on the basis of the experience of the body relating to objects in different orientations

Squinting—Narrowing the opening of one or both eyes in an effort to see better

Symptoms—Subjective descriptions of a problem, such as seeing blurry or double

Strabismus—An eye that turns in toward the nose or out toward the ear

Tactile sense—Having a basic awareness of where and how a person has been touched; also a discriminative touch as a basis for skill building

Tactile defensiveness—Responding to touch as if it were uncomfortable or threatening; this response interferes with relating well to others and can interfere with skill development

Template—A sturdy piece of cardboard with a shape cut out that can be used to guide drawing with chalk or pen on a board or paper

Vestibular system—The sensory system with receptors in the inner ear, which responds to changes in head position to help us keep our balance; this system is constantly "checking in" with our eyes, muscles, and joints to keep us oriented to gravity and to how we balance and move our bodies

Vision—As defined by Dr Gerald Getman, vision enables individuals to gather, analyze, process, store, and respond to light information. It is the ability to understand what is seen. Another definition, from Dr Robert Kraskin, is "the deriving of meaning and directing of action stimulated by light."

Vision therapy—A program or arranged conditions of learning directed toward development of a more efficient and effective visual system; vision therapy is effective for both children and adults

Visual attention—The ability to attend with the visual system; a vital component of total attention

Visual discrimination—The ability to see similarities and differences and to determine whether objects are identical; the ability to see one object and separate it from the background, as in picking out one tree in a forest

Visual motor integration—The ability to put together information from the eyes and other parts of the body (eg, the hands) to perform a task, such as writing or shaking hands; the connection between seeing and doing

Visualization—The ability to see something in the mind's eye

About the Authors

Rebecca Hutchins, OD, FCOVD

Dr Hutchins is a behavioral optometrist who has been in practice in the Boulder, Colorado, area since 1984. She speaks and consults frequently on the behavioral aspects of vision, cortical visual impairment, vision deficits in the gifted and twice exceptional, and evaluation and treatment of visual sequelae after mild traumatic brain injury. She has a particular interest in the nonvisual portion of the optic nerve, the newly discovered photoreceptor melanopsin, and and how the two relate to mood, sleep, and possible links to cancers in individuals who work at night. She believes that working with vision is vital to the whole person and coordinates her care with parents, teachers, other therapists, and tutors.

Lois Hickman, MS, OTR, FAOTA

Lois is an occupational therapist who has been practicing in the Boulder, Colorado, area since 1972. She has practiced in both hospital and clinical settings and has lectured nationally and internationally on sensory integration, the utilization of music and story in occupational therapy, and the application of occupational therapy in therapeutic horseback riding. Currently, her private practice with children and adults has encompassed clinical work, farming, and therapeutic horseback riding. She enjoys collaborating with clients, families, and other professionals on ways to incorporate fun (including musical fun) into the often-serious business of therapy.

"Be the change you want to see in the world."

— Mohandas Gandhi

The authors especially thank Lynn F. Hellerstein, OD, FCOVD, of Centennial, Colorado. Her consultation was invaluable in preparing the information for both the original and updated version of *Eyegames*. Dr Hellerstein has worked with children and adults who exhibit a variety of visual-perceptual challenges. She has also helped athletes improve their skills by fine-tuning the critical connection between vision and motor control. Her most recent book is *See It. Say it. Do it! The Parent's & Teacher's Action Guide to Creating Successful Students and Confident Kids.*

How I Became a Doctor of Optometry

Rebecca E. Hutchins, OD, FCOVD

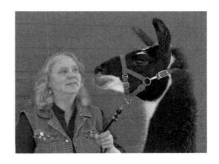

I enjoyed school and was a pretty good student in all subjects except mathematics. I really enjoyed biology in high school, but when I considered pursuing biology in college, I felt that I would not be able to handle the math. I also greatly enjoyed reading and literature, so I went to college and received a bachelor's degree (from Washington College in Chestertown, Maryland) and a master's degree (from American University in Washington, DC) in English literature. I chose to write a thesis for my master's degree, although it was not required, and the title was, "Epigraphs as an Informing Factor to the Poetry of T. S. Eliot." In 1974, when I was writing my thesis, personal computers had not yet been invented. I therefore typed my entire 80-page thesis, in draft and final form, on a typewriter.

I have been near-sighted since the 2nd grade, and at the time I was typing my thesis, I wore hard contact lenses. I was also working part-time as secretary to the medical director of the American Psychiatric Association (APA) in Washington, DC, so most of my waking hours involved "close" work. I began to be unable to finish a page without inverting or reversing several letters on the page. The more tired I became, the more this occurred. Some friends suggested that I visit a behavioral optometrist—I had always received vision care from an ophthalmologist up until this time.

Dr Amiel Francke, from his office on "I" Street, in Washington, DC, explained that my eyes did not work well together—an issue that was separate from my long-standing near-sightedness. I was excited to begin a program of vision therapy with him, aimed at improving my poor visual skills. My boss at the APA, a medical doctor, did not approve of this choice, but I began to work with Dr Francke, and after a short time, I noticed changes not only in the efficiency of my typing, but also in my way of looking at the world. One time, when I asked him why I perceived something the way I do, he said, "You couldn't understand." I took this as a challenge and I went back to school, earning the prerequisites needed to enter optometry school. By this time, I had worked as a computer programmer for a few years, and my boss at the time cautioned me against going back to school, saying, "You'll be thirty-two by the time you get out of school, and you'll be in debt and have a net loss of lifetime income." I countered that I'd be 32 in 4 years' time no matter what, and that I was intrigued with the idea of working more holistically with the visual system.

So at the age of 29, I entered Pennsylvania College of Optometry (now called Salus University), and I not only received an excellent education, but I was able to learn about low vision (an optometric subspecialty) at their Feinbloom Rehabilitation Center. I completed internships at the Gesell Institute for Child Development in New Haven, Connecticut; the Alaska Native Medical Center in Anchorage, Alaska; and a vision therapy office in Boulder, Colorado. In my 3rd year, I wrote a paper for a class in environmental optometry entitled, "The Nonvisual Portion of the Optic Nerve: Implications for the Optometrist." It won the Knight Henry Award in 1984, my senior year, and ironically foreshadowed my current interest in melanopsin, the newly discovered photoreceptor that controls the production of melatonin. I've learned so much in the quarter of a century I've worked in this field, and one of the best experiences has been sharing ideas with like-minded professionals, of which Lois Hickman is probably my favorite. We've shared clients and ideas for all this time, traded animals back and forth, and plan to buy some day-old chicks together very soon.

It's been a strange path for a math-phobic English major—but here I am!

The Journey to JenLo Farm

Lois Hickman, MS, OTR, FAOTA

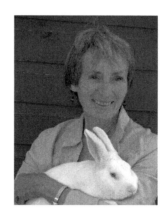

When I was growing up, I lived near aunts and uncles and cousins (within minutes of each other on a "poor-folks'" dirt road, just outside the city limits), where it was often difficult to tell who belonged to whom. The Depression, as well as various family calamities, created a need for everyone to take care of each other. You never knew which cousin's feet would be on your pillow—it all depended on who needed to be taken care of at the time. The trailer in our backyard belonged to an out-of-work family friend, who also happened to be a poet. He was part of our family for 5 years.

When I was young, my father told nightly bedtime stories about "Grandpa Turtle" or "Grandpa Catfish," who warned against hurting their "babies." On my way home from school, I used to take shortcuts through the woods, where I tasted wild strawberries, picked violets, witnessed snakes digesting mice, and nearly lost my boots in the sticky mud in the springtime. I shed angry tears and joined sign-wielding protest marches over a maple tree being cut down in my neighborhood, or over the conversion of a vacant lot (that was "our" softball field) into somebody else's new home. I took art lessons and the begged-for piano lessons.

We also used to make regular pilgrimages to my grandparents' farm in Shepherd, Michigan. The potatoes and beets and carrots harvested there were stored in their root cellar (ah, the musty smell of that root cellar!). The peas, beans, apples, and berries grown on our ⅛ of an acre in Flint, Michigan, joined the Shepherd produce in shining glass canning jars under the stairway to our attic, and they constituted most of our winter fare.

When it came time to decide on a career path, I was presented with a dilemma: music? art? A high-school friend mentioned that she was going to become an occupational therapist. I asked what that was, and when she told me, I immediately knew that occupational therapy was what I wanted to do. I could see the possibility of including *all* my interests in this profession. I earned a BS and an MS in occupational therapy after attending Eastern Michigan University and Colorado State University. Then I became a member of Jean Ayres' faculty, which was grounded in sensory integrative theory. I was fascinated by how all of the senses overlap and influence each other and by how vibration is the basis for all of our senses. This all contributed to my understanding of human development and of ways to reach even the most "involved" clients.

As an occupational therapist, the influence of my childhood experiences became evident. At Boulder Memorial Hospital, treks on the greenbelt outside the hospital grounds were easily woven into therapy sessions. At The Children's Hospital in Denver, a social worker, a speech therapist, and I developed an outward-bound camp experience for children with sensory processing problems at Breckenridge Colorado. There were trips to a local llama farm and to the Denver zoo, as well as backpacking outings around the inner city to meet neighborhood children, hear their stories, and explore the natural environment, which was easy to overlook unless you slowed down to really see it.

Near our clinic in Niwot, Colorado, we hiked on a trail where families of owls graced the ancient cottonwoods. We visited the goat farm only a mile away, sometimes to enjoy hot cocoa made from a stream of goat milk squirted directly into a mug of instant cocoa mix. Ahhh, delicious!

At Stonebridge Farm, near Lyons, Colorado, we began yearly summer camps for children with special needs. And, finally, with the purchase of JenLo Farm (directly west of Stonebridge), therapy for children and adults is blended into the real work of caring for rabbits, pigs, goats, chickens, ducks, fish, dogs, cats, and— at various times—a donkey, a Jersey cow, and a miniature horse. Farm therapy addresses all the issues that are usually thought to belong in a clinic, without the "feel" of a hospital or clinic.

Farm chores and activities encompass movement, touch, strengthening, balance, and practical problem solving. Awareness of the changing seasons is experienced graphically by the changing length of the days, the fruits ripening, the vegetables becoming ready to harvest, and the changing needs of the animals as the days grow warmer or colder. A very important aspect of farm therapy is that, as chores are being done, empathy for "others" evolves through relating to the animals. This is often the bridge that leads to being able to relate to and care for other people.

JenLo Farm is a caring community. Kids don't like to leave—they feel almost as if this farm belongs to them, as they learn where the feed is kept, what kind of care each animal needs, and how the needs on the farm change as the seasons do. Clients develop a respect for life and a love for the natural world. Beyond the farm, our clients are often included when we visit the local hardware or feed store or go to the natural food store, where scraps are saved for the animals. Community awareness and inclusion broadens the influence of therapy on the farm.

Our community has expanded to include friends from around the world. In addition to the many occupational-therapy students from the United States who have undergone internships here, there have been outstanding students from Japan and Ireland. I have conducted workshops in Japan, South Africa, and Scotland on the importance of incorporating music and story into therapy sessions and on the value of conducting occupational therapy in a natural setting—including therapeutic horseback riding.

The environment of JenLo Farm suits me well. I live where I work. At the end of the day, there may be feet on my pillow, but now, instead of cousins, they're apt to belong to a dog, a cat, a crippled chicken, or even a duck. What can I say—it's a good life.

Resources

There are many excellent products and reference materials available from the following organizations.

Sensory World
721 W Abram St
Arlington, TX 76013
Phone: (800) 489-0727 or (817) 277-0727
Fax: (817) 277-2270
info@sensoryworld.com
www.sensoryworld.com

Sensory World, a proud division of Future Horizons, is the world's largest publisher devoted exclusively to resources for those interested in sensory processing disorder. They also sponsor national conferences for parents, teachers, therapists, and others interested in supporting those with sensory processing disorder. Visit *www.sensoryworld.com* for further information.

Sensory products include *Answers to Questions Teachers Ask About Sensory Intgration, The Goodenoughs Get in Sync, The Sensory Connection, Prechool SENSE, Starting SI Therapy, MoveAbout Cards, 28 Instant Songames, Songames for Sensory Integration, Danceland, Marvelous Mouth Music, The Out-of-Sync Child* video, *Making Sense of Sensory Integration, Teachers Ask about Sensory Integration, Eyegames,* and *Soothing the Senses.*

American Occupational Therapy Association
4720 Montgomery Lane
Bethesda, MD 20824-1220
Phone: (301) 652-2682 or (800) 377-8555
Fax: (301) 652-7711

College of Optometrists and Vision Development
215 West Garfield Rd, Ste 200
Aurora, OH 44202
Phone: (330) 995-0718 or (888) 268-3770
Fax: (339) 995-9719
www.covd.org

The College of Optometrists and Vision Development provides excellent information on all aspects of vision.

Developmental Delay Resources
5801 Beacon St
Pittsburgh, PA 15217
Phone: (800) 497-0944
Fax: (412) 422-1374
www.devdelay.org

Developmental Delay Resources publishes the quarterly newsletter *New Developments,* sponsors workshops, and is a clearinghouse on alternative approaches regarding educational and medical concerns of children with special needs.

Optometric Extension Program Foundation
1921 E Carnegie Ave, Ste 3L
Santa Ana, CA 92705-5510
Phone: (949) 250-8070
www.oep.org

The Optometric Extension Program Foundation provides products, information, and workshops relating to improving visual motor skills.